Distribution, publication, and copying in any form are prohibited and subject to damages.

TEN HYPNOSES

Copying, publishing, and sharing with third parties are only permitted with the written consent of the author. Please observe the notes on copyright and usage.

Distribution, publication, and copying in any form are prohibited and subject to damages.

Copying, publishing, and sharing with third parties are only permitted with the written consent of the author. Please observe the notes on copyright and usage.

Ingo Michael Simon

TEN HYPNOSES

33

Fear of Illness, Hypochondria

Distribution, publication, and copying in any form are prohibited and subject to damages.

© 2024 Ingo Michael Simon
All rights reserved.
Independently published
www.ingosimon.com

Important Notes for Urgent Attention:

The contents of this book are based on the practical experiences of the author with hypnosis applications and psychotherapy in a trance state. Although the author has strived for the utmost care, errors or misunderstandings in the presentation cannot be completely excluded. Therapeutic work with people and the application of hypnosis are solely the responsibility of the hypnotist. It cannot be ruled out that parts of this book may be misunderstood or that the application of a presented procedure may cause an undesirable reaction in the client. The author also assumes no co-responsibility if work with a client is carried out with reference to the statements in this book.

The Author:

Ingo Michael Simon studied psychology and education and is a hypnotherapist with practices in southwestern Germany and Switzerland. With the help of hypnosis-supported psychotherapy, he primarily treats people with persistent psychological conditions. His practice focuses on anxiety disorders, pathological compulsions, and psychosomatic illnesses. His therapeutic offerings mainly include classical and modern hypnosis applications and the dreamland therapy he developed himself.

Copying, publishing, and sharing with third parties are only permitted with the written consent of the author. Please observe the notes on copyright and usage.

Distribution, publication, and copying in any form are prohibited and subject to damages.

INTRODUCTION	**6**
COPYRIGHT AND USAGE	**8**
HYPNOSIS 1	**10**
HYPNOSIS 2	**15**
HYPNOSIS 3	**20**
HYPNOSIS 4	**25**
HYPNOSIS 5	**29**
HYPNOSIS 6	**33**
HYPNOSIS 7	**37**
HYPNOSIS 8	**42**
HYPNOSIS 9	**48**
HYPNOSIS 10	**53**
ALL TITLES IN THE SERIES	**58**

Copying, publishing, and sharing with third parties are only permitted with the written consent of the author. Please observe the notes on copyright and usage.

Introduction

The series "Ten Hypnoses" is very well known in Germany, Austria, and Switzerland as a collection of texts for therapeutic work and is used by numerous psychotherapeutic practices, doctors, therapists, coaches, and other helping professionals. I am pleased to now be able to offer these texts in other countries as well.

Most therapists have their own methods for inducing and deepening trance as well as for exiting trance. Therefore, I have focused on the main part of the hypnosis. The texts in this book can be integrated as the main part into any hypnosis process. The texts in this collection use various hypnosis techniques. I will not explain these in detail, as I assume that users have the appropriate training. It is also not necessary to understand the exact structure or functioning of the different parts. The texts can simply be read aloud, and they will have their effect.

Decide for yourself which text best suits your client or patient at any given time. You can also combine passages from different texts. It is not about using all ten hypnoses in sequence. It is a selection of possibilities.

I want to emphasize that books cannot replace therapy. Psychotherapy or other therapeutic treatments involve much more. A careful diagnosis is the necessary basis for deciding on the use of methods, including whether hypnosis or one of my texts should be used. Even in this case, preparatory discussions, follow-up discussions during the session, and of course, a therapeutic concept for the sequence of sessions and the content approaches are essential parts of therapy. This cannot and should not be achieved with a collection of texts.

In any case, I wish you much success in your work and I am pleased if my text templates can contribute in a small way.

Ingo Michael Simon

Copyright and Usage

Copying, publishing, and sharing with third parties is prohibited and only permitted with the written consent of the author. Please observe the following copyright and usage guidelines.

This work has been carefully crafted and created to the best of the author's knowledge and personal experience. It comprises text templates and application guidelines for professional hypnosis sessions. The author is a licensed psychotherapist with extensive experience in psychotherapy, coaching, and personal training using hypnotic techniques and methods. Nevertheless, the author and the publisher assume no liability for the accuracy of information, instructions, and advice, nor for any typographical errors. The author and publisher accept no responsibility or liability for the application of these texts and recommendations with clients or patients, nor for any potential consequences or unexpected reactions. It is expressly noted that the application of therapeutic and advisory techniques and formulations lies solely and entirely within the responsibility of the practitioner. This also applies to adherence to the boundaries of legally regulated medical and therapeutic practices. The fact that a book containing action proposals is freely available for sale does not imply that its application with clients or patients is permitted for everyone.

Hypnosis 1

You know that you are healthy... You are familiar with the exaggerated fear of illness and have realized that it is unnecessary... So, you want to let go of the fear of diseases... You are determined and ready to release the fear of infections and illnesses today... You are already succeeding in letting go of this fear today... You succeed because you truly understand that a slight twinge or itch is completely normal... You know that the feelings and sensations in your body are entirely normal... You are fully aware that your body sends you friendly signals... These small signals show you that your body is alert and attentive... and that's why it's healthy... because it takes care of itself and of you... Your body is healthy... You are healthy... You are truly healthy, and you know it... and that's why you free yourself from fear today...

You know that positive thoughts can help you repeatedly recognize that you are indeed healthy... and only visit a doctor if it's genuinely necessary... Positive thoughts help you... They help you stay calm and relaxed when you feel a twinge or pressure somewhere... Constructive thoughts help you realize that the fear of illness is completely exaggerated... You have often thought you might be ill... or knew you were healthy but felt an unease that you didn't understand... Calmness helps you... Calmness and clarity help you... You construct your health-focused thoughts... You tell yourself... I feel free and healthy, I am well... You are thinking this thought now... That is enough... because now, in this pleasant trance, this thought is deeply ingrained and becomes a fundamental attitude... because this thought reflects the truth... You are free... You are healthy... You feel good...

Your bodily awareness helps you repeatedly recognize that you are healthy... continually distinguishing between healthy, normal sensations and those that might indicate illness... But above all, your bodily awareness is important at this moment... the feeling you have now... Your body feels healthy now... You are calm inside and can become even more relaxed... You feel comfortable... Your heart beats calmly and steadily... Your circulation is stable... Your organs function like clockwork... You are healthy... You can feel it clearly... Now you can clearly feel that you are healthy... All the functions of your body and organs are in order... Even when you focus entirely on how your body feels, you can see that you are indeed healthy... Your body can learn again to clearly signal this healthy state to you... especially when you might think you could be ill... From now on, your body helps you stay calm and relaxed...

Fear is a feeling... The fear of illness or being ill is a feeling... Calmness is also a feeling... Calmness and serenity are feelings... Calmness or fear... Only one can exist at a time... Now you feel calm inside, and you are relaxed... and therefore, you cannot feel fear now... Focus your mindfulness and attention on the feeling of calmness within you... This sense of calm becomes clearer now... You grow calmer with each breath... Your calmness deepens... Every moment of conscious calmness and relaxation dissolves fearful expectations and thoughts... Every moment of conscious calmness and relaxation strengthens the feeling of being healthy... You build new trust in your healthy body... because you truly have one... a healthy body... You can feel it... You are healthy... Your body is healthy and strong... You are confident that you are healthy... and that's why you let go of anxious thoughts and feel good about it... You are once again sure that you are truly healthy… You are completely sure that your body is healthy… and will remain healthy…

You resolve to do something so that you can always let go of fearful thoughts and immediately return to inner calm and serenity… You are already succeeding today… You let go of the fear of infection or illness today… You free yourself from fear… You free yourself from all worries… Whenever you might even begin to sense any worries, you shift into your new helpful thought, and it becomes true… I feel free and healthy, I am well… This thought immediately becomes true… because calmness and fear cannot exist at the same time… Your calm thought takes center stage… Your new thought expands further and further… and fear fades away… Fear must fade because calmness spreads… Whenever a thought of fear might arise, you say… I feel free and healthy, I am well… and immediately you feel your body relax and calm down with this thought… and you can clearly feel how your body really feels…

You are once again sure that your body is healthy… You are once again sure that you are healthy… You feel what your thought says… I feel free and healthy, I am well… This health-focused thought helps you feel free every day... You feel good... Your heart beats calmly and steadily... Your organs function perfectly... Every day, you can feel free because you let go of fear... and therefore, you feel free and healthy... free and healthy every day... You experience freedom and health every day...

Hypnosis 2

Today, you focus on the signals your body sends you... You have often felt sensations that you interpreted as signs of illness, but you know that you were and are healthy... So, today, you want to recalibrate your perception... You want to be able to quickly distinguish between bodily signals that are indeed signs of illness and those sensations that are normal and completely harmless... (1) You concentrate on your goal of intuitively and calmly sensing your body again and understanding what each sensation means... (2) Today, you are already succeeding in distinguishing between the usual sensations of your body and actual signs of illness... (3) Today, you are resetting your body... like an inner adjustment... Your self-awareness is once again following your natural instinct, allowing you to recognize normal sensations as harmless... and you can see every day that most of your body's perceptions and sensations are just regular and ordinary sensations... which might be caused by digestion, breathing, or other completely ordinary processes in the body...

Now you realize that you can truly achieve this goal today... You remember that you have already achieved many goals in your life... and that you used to be calm and carefree... Again and again, there were challenges in your life that you embraced... (1) Most often, it was your own potential that enabled you to take on challenges successfully... Just as it is today... You are successful again today... (2) You already succeed today... You are indeed capable of leaving the fear of illness behind... simply ending it and then feeling that you are healthy again... (3) More is possible today than ever before, because today is the right time for a change... Today is the right moment to recognize and clearly feel that you are healthy... So today, calmness replaces the fear you once felt... and you feel that your body feels good... You can recognize the usual sensations of your body and stay calm and relaxed because everything is fine... You are healthy...

First, we internally separate the fears of illness, as they are exaggerated... You can also achieve this with your own potential... with your potential for overcoming and letting go... You had this before... you have often used your potential for life's challenges... (1) Deep inside, at this very moment, you feel relaxation and with it calmness and serenity... Calmness and serenity that help you understand your body's sensations correctly... Now, at this very moment, your body feels healthy... because you feel healthy, and you are relaxed... with your eyes closed, you can feel your body even more clearly than when fully awake... and you feel that everything is in order... Your body feels good... (2) There are no worries right now... You are calm and relaxed... much calmer than usual... Even when thinking about potential illnesses, you remain calm... (3) All the sensations of your body are entirely ordinary and normal now... whatever you feel or sense right now... it is normal, and you are healthy... normal and healthy... (1) You let go of all worries about illnesses now... (2) You truly let go of all worries now... You are healthy, and therefore you are also calm... (3) Now you even let go of the memory of worrying about illnesses, so that they cannot come back... Now, at this moment, you let go of everything connected to the fear of infection and illness...

Imagine something very beautiful... a truly beautiful memory or a wonderful fantasy... (1) Now, positive and beautiful thoughts flow through your entire body... (2) Now, more and more beautiful thoughts flood through you... Thoughts that are so lovely that there is no room for illness... beautiful thoughts of calmness... beautiful thoughts of serenity... (3) The most beautiful thoughts you can imagine spread throughout you... Now, only these beautiful thoughts matter, creating a new connection... Imagine the most beautiful memory... or the most beautiful moment... or the most beautiful fantasy... And with this beautiful thought, a new connection is formed... Serenity within you... Serenity in your thoughts... Serenity in your feelings... Serenity within you...

(1) You have done it... Amazing how quickly you can adapt and have already distanced yourself from the fear of illness... (2) Truly amazing and really strong because you have done it... you have distanced yourself far from the fear of infection and illness... very far... (3) You have already let go of the old fears of infection and illness... You have internally separated from the old fear and then let it go... That is a big step... the most important step... a real accomplishment... well done... very, very well done...

Now you can rest because you have achieved a lot... Maybe you feel surprisingly fit and full of energy... Perhaps this quick change did not seem very strenuous to you... Maybe it was really easy for you to follow this trance... It may have been effortless for you to follow my words... because you have been preparing yourself to let go of the old fear for a long time and only needed a small step... a gentle push... You have freed yourself... freed from fear... You are healthy... normal and healthy... normal and healthy...

Hypnosis 3

You have decided to end the fear of illness... to first detach from it and then let it disappear completely... You know that fear has been holding you... Fear when thinking about possible illnesses, fear when noticing small bodily sensations... a slight twinge or harmless sounds in the stomach... You also know the anticipatory fear that could start even before any actual perception... Let's call all these exaggerated fears related to infections and illnesses simply "illness anxiety"... It is a fear, so it's a feeling... Feelings manifest in our body and our thoughts... So today, you can use your body's perception and your body's feelings to end the illness anxiety... That is possible... It is really possible, and it happens today... It happens today... It happens today...

You have often intensely perceived your body, paying close attention to what feelings you could sense and then interpreted them as signs of illness... You know that these were exaggerated interpretations because you were healthy... But then thoughts and worries kept coming back, thinking that maybe something was wrong... Today you can do it differently... Today, you can consciously and intensely perceive your body and feel it while being certain that you are healthy... In trance, this is possible... In trance, it's even easy... You are healthy, and you know it... Feel your body, you are healthy... Feel your body, perceive it clearly now, you are healthy... Go from head to toe along your body as if with a scanner that slowly moves from your head to your feet... and feel that you can consciously perceive your body... Consciously perceive your body with every sensation that might be there... Whatever you feel, let it be, because these are natural and normal bodily sensations within you... You are healthy... Feel your body, you are healthy... Perceive every movement of your body, you are healthy... Let every sensation become clear, you are healthy... You are healthy, and you know it... You are healthy, and you are completely sure that you are healthy and will remain healthy... You let go of the fear... It happens today... It happens now... Now... Whatever you feel and perceive now... You are healthy and let go of the fear... It happens today... It happens now... Now...

You find the part of your body where you most often feared there was an illness... maybe somewhere in your abdomen or chest... Perhaps it was often your heart that you thought was sick... or a completely different part... You find the part of your body that you often suspected... Now you know that you are healthy... Now you know that everything is okay... Everything is really okay because you are healthy... Whatever you feel at this particular spot now, you are healthy... But there are also parts of your body where you never suspected an illness... Now you find a part of your body that has always been healthy... maybe a hand or a finger... or a foot, who knows... You find a part of your body that you have always experienced as healthy... There you have never felt a strange twinge or sting, never a signal that you couldn't quite place... Your full attention goes to this spot... You have always experienced health there... Everything has always been okay there... So it is now... That's how a healthy body feels... This is exactly how being healthy feels... Imagine that these two parts of your body are connected... and from the always healthy part of your body, the feeling of health flows to the part you often thought was sick... Both areas are connected, and both feel healthy... Imagine this connection like a bridge... a bridge over which healthy warmth flows... healthy warmth within you... and this warmth now spreads throughout your entire body... From the always healthy part of your body, pleasant and healthy warmth flows like a healing breeze through your entire body... your whole being is flooded with healing warmth... You feel that this health is spreading throughout your body... You are completely healthy... Every possible worry about infection and illness is dissolved and replaced by health... It happens today... It happens now... It happens today... It happens now...

And once again, you go along your body as if with a scanner, to feel that you can indeed sense health everywhere... Start at your head and slowly move down to your feet... and everywhere you once suspected or feared illness, maybe even just half an hour ago, you discover relaxation and calmness and health... And if there is still any doubt somewhere, stay focused there until you can feel the warmth there too and are sure you can feel health... Well done... You're doing it right... You're succeeding...

Keep breathing calmly and steadily and trust that with each breath, your body spreads more health and further dissolves and eliminates illness anxiety... especially when you are awake again, because then your subconscious has time and opportunity to continue dissolving the illness anxiety... filling your body with healing warmth and truly resolving the illness anxiety... It happens today... It happens now...

Hypnosis 4

Today, you want to end the fear of illness and infection... It works because it's a feeling that once served a purpose but no longer fits... You have no use for this fear anymore... It's a relic from a past time... Somehow it got stuck, but now it's time to end it and finally allow calmness and relaxation to return... It's time again to enjoy the day and be completely relaxed with yourself and your health... Your body is fine... Your body is healthy... You can use a thought that restores normality...

Imagine lying in a hammock and falling asleep... It's a beautiful, warm day, and you've fallen asleep peacefully, dreaming a lovely dream... maybe a beautiful memory, or you're dreaming of an upcoming experience that you imagine as wonderful... and with the images in your dream come pleasant, beautiful feelings... Maybe you've heard that we only dream feelings... and the dream images we see are representations that match our feelings in the dream... So you dream beautiful images because you've found beautiful feelings deep inside... Perhaps your hammock sways a bit back and forth... and back... and forth... back... and forth... and more and more beautiful images suddenly appear before your inner eye... They are just there, and you repeatedly feel pleasant feelings... Let yourself drift in your lovely dream, which is a dream of lightness and serenity... a dream of health...

Then you wake up and open your eyes, looking directly at the bright blue sky... You wake up with the beautiful feelings from your dream... You dreamed so wonderfully that you wake up with a very nice feeling... still feeling good and sleepily realizing that it's still daylight... You look up at the bright blue summer sky and see writing in thick letters in the sky... You can clearly see it, you can read it because it's your thought that is written there... Up there in the bright blue sky is written what you know deep inside... what you believe deep inside... Up there, in thick letters, it says...

I trust in my body's self-regulation and recognize that I am healthy.

Then you think about how often you thought you might be sick, but your body was healthy... Your body's self-regulation is working... and when you were actually sick, it felt different... Then you knew it for sure... but in doubt, you were always healthy... So you let the words you read in the sky resonate within you... let them become a feeling deep inside... and this feeling within you gives you beautiful dreams again... Important words become normality... and the words you read in the sky become normality within you... Now... your normality, the normality of your feelings... Now... You fall asleep again, and your beautiful dreams become even more beautiful... It is this thought that makes your dreams so beautiful... that leads you back to the normality of serenity in dealing with yourself... It is this affirmation that you can think or speak over and over again... It is this normality that you can recognize over and over again... that becomes your inner wisdom... a deep belief that helps you recognize normal bodily sensations and remain calm and serene... as calm as you are now... just as calm and serene as you are now...

Deep within you, these words become ingrained as normality. They help you recognize again and again that you are healthy... Once again, the words you hear have an effect...

I trust in my body's self-regulation and recognize that I am healthy.

... These special words have a deep effect and help you recognize again and again that you are healthy when you are indeed healthy... Today, deep inside, you are relearning to clearly distinguish when you are sick and when you are healthy... You can recognize both accurately when these words have a deep effect...

The affirmation you heard helps you live in harmony with your body again... so that you can be in harmony with your perception and sensations again and always clearly recognize what your body is actually signaling to you... You once again recognize the everyday nature and normality of your bodily sensations... And you experience all ordinary sensations with calmness...

Hypnosis 5

You have a goal, and you are determined to achieve it today... It is a special goal... You want to feel free again, let go of the fear of illness... and enjoy every day without worry... You have experienced the fear of infection and illness... But that fear should end today... The fear should end today... because now you can align yourself internally with freedom and health again... You can feel free again and enjoy every day anew... You trust your healthy body again... Today, you can use the trance to do that... You are in trance now... and that's why it's possible to find help deep within yourself... deep inside, in the unconscious... Now, you are free from fear... Now, you are also free enough to talk to your subconscious... and your subconscious accepts all your suggestions and implements them for you... Now... So you say...

... I recognize that I am healthy and safe... because I am aware that I am strong and grown-up... ... I recognize that I am healthy and safe... because I know that I don't need to fear illnesses... ... I recognize that I am healthy and safe...

because I have been healthy and safe for the past years/months... ... I recognize that I am healthy and safe... because the fact that I am healthy is true... ... I am healthy... I am truly healthy...

... I recognize my body's signals as natural and healthy reactions... because they show me that my body is active and all my organs are working reliably... ... I recognize my body's signals as natural and healthy reactions... because with them, my body shows me that everything is fine... ... I recognize my body's signals as natural and healthy reactions... because with them, my body shows me that all my organs are functioning and doing their job... ... I recognize my body's signals as natural and healthy reactions... because a healthy body can only show healthy reactions... ... I am healthy... I am truly healthy...

... I am confident that my body maintains its health... that's also why I can let go of fear... ... I am confident that my body maintains its health... that's also why I can clearly recognize that I am healthy... ... I am confident that my body maintains its health... that's also why I can be open and curious again... ... I am confident that my body maintains its health... that's also why I am sure that I am truly healthy and will stay healthy... ... I am healthy... I am truly healthy...

... I feel calm and relaxed, I feel free... because I have realized that fear of illness is exaggerated... ... I feel calm and relaxed, I feel free... because I have realized that I would clearly feel if I were ill... ... I feel calm and relaxed, I feel free... because I have realized that most bodily signals are ordinary reactions of my healthy body... ... I feel calm and relaxed, I feel free... because I have realized that I am indeed free and healthy inside... ... I am healthy... I am truly healthy...

... I enjoy each new day with relaxation and joy... because I know that I am truly healthy... ... I enjoy each new day with relaxation and joy... because I know that I will stay truly healthy... ... I enjoy each new day with relaxation and joy... because I know that each day offers so much beauty... ... I enjoy each new day with relaxation and joy... because I know that with free thoughts, I can enjoy life even more... ... I am healthy... I am truly healthy... [30 seconds of silence]...

Alright... You have done the most important part... Now let all the words you've heard flow deep into your inner self... into your subconscious... because there they become truth... Deep inside, they are already the truth... Everything you have heard becomes what you say... Everything you say becomes a deep belief... a deep truth... You know deep inside that you are completely healthy... and that's exactly what you can feel again... You feel that you are truly healthy... You are and will remain healthy...

Hypnosis 6

You know the fear of infection and illness and have often believed you were sick... Then it turned out that your fears were exaggerated and false... You were healthy, and you are healthy... You want to recognize again that you are healthy... You want to be free in your thoughts so that you don't even have these troubling thoughts in the first place... So today, you enter into a special connection with yourself... different than usual... You have tried to fight against the worries about illness... Today, you do it differently... Today, you turn to your body and thank it for functioning so well... You speak to your body... Let my words become your words... and say...

Dear body... I want to thank you today... for serving me so well and so patiently all these years... I know that you have mostly been healthy and that because of that, I have mostly been healthy too... Often, I thought you were sick, but I know that in truth, you were healthy... You continued to function even when I thought you were sick... I thank my bones... for holding me up and allowing me to move... I also thank all my muscles and tendons... because they, too, contribute to me moving healthily and powerfully... I know it's a teamwork... that bones, tendons, and muscles work together for me... Today, I also thank all my internal organs... Through their work, they provide my body with nutrients and keep it healthy... It is also the internal organs that detoxify the body and keep me healthy again and again... Often, I thought that some of these organs were sick, but I know that they were always healthy and worked well for me... For that, I sincerely thank all my internal organs today... I also thank my heart, which has always worked well for me... even and especially when I thought my heart was sick or beating too fast or irregularly... It continued its faithful service steadily, and for that, I thank my heart today... my own heart... I also thank my feet, which have always carried the weight of my whole body... and I thank my hands, which have always had to grip and grasp... And I especially thank all the many little helpers in my body... the many small organs and components that work together like clockwork every day... to keep my body healthy and functioning well... And finally, I also thank my head, which is the control center of my body... I thank my head and my brain for perfectly controlling and regulating my entire body… for making sure that all parts always work well together and do so every day… Dear body, I thank you for that today…

Dear body… Please help me also to recognize more quickly from now on that you are healthy… especially when I feel a twinge or some other sensation that I cannot immediately identify… You have always helped me; please help me with this too… Every day, I want to remember that you have always helped me… and that's why I trust that with your support, I can truly let go of the fear of illness…

Dear body… I know that I need to take care of my inner feelings, my mood, and my deep concerns… the emotions that have nothing to do with you but only with me… Dear body… I ask for your support in being patient with myself if I don't immediately succeed in freeing myself from fear… because with your help, I will succeed in the end… with your help, I will truly be free from fear and deeply feel that I am healthy…

Dear body… Today, I want to start being patient and considerate with myself… I treat myself with self-love, and I ask for help in truly being able to accept myself... in really feeling the sense of self-love... With your help, I will succeed even more quickly and clearly in embracing myself with love... Dear body... I trust in your help and thank you for your guidance and support on my journey to freedom...

Well done... Now you may rest... Trust that a part of you has accepted these words as your own... and your body, as part of you, has listened as a helper and will help you achieve your goal... You let go of the fear of illness... You feel healthy... You are healthy... You are truly healthy...

Hypnosis 7

You want to end the exaggerated fear of infection and illness today... You know that you didn't have this fear before, and that's why you can be free from it again... Today, you take an inner journey through time to rediscover that time of freedom from fear... But this journey is more than a journey through time... It's a journey through your feelings, because within you, there is still that calmness and serenity from back then, that natural way of dealing with your body... On your journey, you find that time and that freedom again today...

Think about the time before the illness anxiety... There was this time before the fear because you weren't born with such fear... You can return to that time... Today, it's possible... as an inner journey... as a journey in thoughts and feelings... Maybe you know when the fear started... Maybe you can't exactly remember when the fear of infection and illness began... It might have been a slow transition... Imagine standing on a line that is like a timeline... a timeline... You look down and see the number of your age... There's the number... [insert client's age]... This is the present moment... Then close your eyes and mentally step backward on your timeline... and with each step, a year passes... and at the same time, you feel freer with each step... The further back you go, the closer you get to the time without illness anxiety... With each step, you get closer to the time when you were still calm and only thought about illness when you really felt clear symptoms because you could very well recognize when you were actually sick... Perhaps you've already arrived at a time free of anxiety... but on your inner journey along your timeline, you can go even further back... many years... So go further back if it helps you and find a time when you were still completely relaxed with your body and your health... a time when you could clearly recognize when you were healthy and when you were getting sick... and as soon as you arrive at that time, you stop to feel the inner freedom even more clearly... You stop and feel that on your inner journey, you are truly in the time when you didn't know any exaggerated worries about illness... You look down at the timeline and see the number there... maybe a two-digit number or even a single-digit one because you've traveled far back... You recognize on the timeline how old you were... Back then, you didn't know any exaggerated worries... You knew that you were healthy...

Now be watchful and attentive and feel what you feel deep inside... Pay attention to your healthy body sensation, which signals calmness and serenity to you... security and protection and health... and pay attention to your mood... to the feeling of calmness... Illness anxiety is no longer possible now because you are calm inside and out... So now you can only feel calmness... Now, even thinking about possible illnesses is bearable and lets you remain calm... That's how it was back then... That's how it was before the time of fear, and that's exactly where you are now... in the time before illness anxiety... Back then, you didn't have an exaggerated fear of illness... back then, you had exactly this good feeling that you feel now... You are back on the timeline of your life, in the exact time before the fear... You remember... That's how it was before... That's how it is now because you are now internally in that time... because you are in that anxiety-free time... in your feelings, you are there... really...

And with this feeling of freedom inside you, you walk with your eyes closed along the timeline into the future... Just as the timeline took you back, it also leads you into the future... Step by step, straight ahead... So start walking... year by year... Imagine how you walk into the future with this feeling of freedom from back then, which you are now really feeling... beyond today, you walk into the future with this feeling of freedom... with calmness and serenity and completely free from any conceivable worry along the timeline... you come into the near future... maybe a few weeks or months ahead and feel within yourself... You are still free from fear... You are in the future and feel as free as you did before... You don't feel it now... and now you are in the future... without the fear... You open your eyes and look at the timeline... There, you see your age; there it says... [insert client's age]... because you've only traveled a few days or weeks into the future and are truly free from fear there... You have let go of the fear now and replaced it with earlier feelings of freedom and serenity... That's how it is, and that's how it stays...

And so you can return to the present with this feeling of freedom and without fear... completely free from fear and with a good feeling in the present... in the present of today... You walk back along the timeline to today... Just take a few steps back with open eyes and bring calmness and naturalness with you because you have found them again... You have found freedom within you... You were free from fear before... You are free from fear in the future, and you are also free from fear in the present... You arrive on today's date... You are free... free from fear, and you are calm...

Hypnosis 8

Guidelines for Conducting

In this hypnosis session, ideomotor responses are used. Ideomotor responses refer to the phenomenon where our body's movements follow our feelings and thoughts. In everyday life, this response is shown in posture, muscle tension, and movement patterns, which naturally change with mood and thoughts. In trance, ideomotor signals can be used to gather information that the client may not actively communicate. For example, the subconscious can answer questions with an agreed-upon finger signal. Naturally, ideomotor responses can also be used suggestively, such as with arm levitations and catalepsies. An ideomotor approach strengthens trust in hypnosis and in one's ability to change, thus supporting therapy.

+++ End of Guidelines +++

You want to dissolve the exaggerated fear of illness... at least for it to be reduced today and eventually disappear altogether... That's possible because a special part of you is capable of doing that... a part of you that you cannot easily command or contact in your waking state... but in trance, this is possible, because in trance, you are stronger and more connected with yourself; you can directly address and instruct your subconscious... Maybe you already know that your fear is a signal from your subconscious... It has nothing to do with illness; it's just meant to make you pay attention... The fear is like a signal meant to show you that you need to take care of yourself... So, it's not about fear of illness at all... It's an invitation from your subconscious... and today, you follow that invitation...

You connect with your subconscious, and I speak with it... That is possible... It's even easier than you might think... Your subconscious just wants you to connect with it, because then the fear can end... This special part of you, the unconscious or subconscious, won't need to send signals anymore... no more fear...

I need to speak directly with your subconscious for that... Dream in beautiful images, imagine a wonderful landscape, as vividly as possible... and stay in these beautiful images of this landscape... so beautiful that you'd love to be there...

You can hear every word and feel everything, but stay in your beautiful images and imagine that all thoughts and visions, all beautiful images you think of, move to the left side of your body... and you, subconscious of ... [client's name]... come to the right and control the right hand... and give me a signal with a finger on the right hand as soon as you manage to take control of the hand... While the waking mind dreams on the left in beautiful images, you, subconscious of ... [client's name]... come to the right and move a finger on the right hand...

... [Please be patient and keep going. Don't worry—finger signals almost always work! Repeat the prompt a few times kindly and firmly, exuding confidence. If you are sure a finger signal will come, it will happen faster than if you doubt it.] ...

... There's the signal, well done... thank you very much... Now, subconscious of ... [client's name]... make sure that the waking mind dreams deeply on the left side, so that we can work well together... The finger you used to greet me will be the yes finger... You can move it for each confirmation... For rejection, you can move a different finger... But now we want to do what your goal is... Understand the fear of illness and then end it... Let's begin...

Subconscious of ... [client's name]... we really want to try to understand the fear better so that you can then truly end it... because I know that you can and will do it if we handle it carefully... I will ask you some questions, which you can answer with your fingers. For yes, please use the yes finger, and for no, choose a different finger... I'll start asking...

... Does the fear of illness still serve a helpful function for you today?... ... if yes... Then make sure this function flows into the waking mind... ... if no... That's good because it makes it much easier to end the fear...

... Was the fear useful when it first arose?... ... if yes... That was a long time ago; today, you can proceed differently and end the fear... ... if no... Then the fear belongs to the past and you can let it go...

... Is there a connection to childhood and events from back then?... ... if yes... Then we will work on childhood memories later; today, you are already an adult and don't need childhood fears anymore... ... if no... Excellent, it's an issue that hasn't been around for long. You can let go of the fear even faster...

... Is there something about the fear of illness that we haven't yet understood?... ... if yes... We need a new approach to truly understand it together. The fear isn't helping us anymore. We need something different... ... if no... Then we've already discussed what's important to you... Let's look at it further and work on it without fear. Fear is no longer required... End the fear...

... Subconscious of ... [client's name]... You see that we are making a joint effort to understand and help you... The waking mind and I... And we will continue to do that, and I promise you that the waking mind will continue to try to understand your signals and messages...

That's what the waking mind does for you... What you need to do is turn off the fear. Only use fear briefly if there's no other option... Do we agree? ... [No is not an option here] ... Good, then reduce the fear now, take care of everything so that it disappears as much as possible within the next 24 hours, and show me with the yes finger as soon as you're done... [Wait for yes finger]...

Well done, it worked... Now the fear can disappear... Maybe you already feel it, and it's already happening, or you will be happy in the next 24 hours that your thoughts and feelings are free again... really free...

Hypnosis 9

Guidelines for Conducting

In this hypnosis session, a self-hypnosis trigger is established. A self-hypnosis trigger is a signal that initiates the state of trance. With its help, even an inexperienced client can continue working with self-hypnosis at home. Naturally, they can work with simple suggestions they can easily remember and that we should prepare, or they can work with simple visualizations. Triggered self-hypnosis is an excellent tool to give the client a task and to support therapy. This way, the time between sessions at the practice isn't without therapy but is continued at home. Fully self-directed self-hypnosis, without a trigger, can also be learned well but requires a lot of time and practice. Establishing the trigger is a relatively simple task and naturally relieves the client, as I don't want to burden them with training fully self-directed self-hypnosis. Despite all the skepticism, I insist that it's really not a problem to teach a client simple trigger self-hypnosis. It's no more dangerous than meditation or autogenic training or yoga. People survive those just fine at home. I've had numerous patients in my practice who not only managed well with self-hypnosis but also enjoyed it. And if a patient enjoys doing self-hypnosis, no matter how simple the suggestion may be, it is a very good support for compliance. Discuss the process once before the hypnosis and give the client a brief, bullet-point list of the steps of self-hypnosis, so they have a small guide.

+++ End of Guidelines +++

Today, you can train in self-hypnosis... I'll show you how to do it, and then you can use self-hypnosis anytime you want to feel freer and freer... to free yourself from any fear of illness... because with self-hypnosis, it's even easier to let go of fear and feel free... You can do self-hypnosis at any time and as often as you like... Every self-hypnosis session helps you feel free permanently... Now focus on the inner calm you feel, on the state of trance you are in now... This is what self-hypnosis feels like too... completely relaxed and at the same time completely normal... a state you can reach every day... It's easy, and it's completely safe... because you're learning how to do it now... You can decide when and where to go into a beautiful and liberating trance... Isn't that wonderful?... Feel your relaxation clearly now... Feel how good it feels to be in trance now...

Now you're learning to reach the trance state on your own... You can go into trance at home with this too... You use a special word for this, just for you... You use your self-hypnosis trigger... It's called... Iamon... [Emphasize the word, please, on the I... I-amon.]... Make yourself comfortable at home, close your eyes just like here... and then whisper this trigger over and over again until it makes you really tired, which happens very quickly... After just a few repetitions of the trigger, you'll already feel tired... So whisper... Iamon – Iamon – Iamon – Iamon – Iamon – Iamon... and as you do, a lovely trance truly begins to form... maybe just as deep as here... But a light trance is already more than enough... Your trigger Iamon is now deeply ingrained in your unconscious... So you can simply use it whenever you want to go into trance...

Then you need to deepen your trance... You do this by whispering ten times... I relax and let go... You simply whisper... I relax once and let go... I relax twice and let go... I relax three times and let go... and so on... until you finally reach ten and whisper... I relax ten times and let go... and as you do, you go into a beautiful, deep state of relaxation... A part of you goes into a truly beautiful, deep trance, and another part stays awake and steers your trance... You are completely safe...

Then you continue with the main part, which is the most important part of your self-hypnosis... You work in this part with a suggestion that frees you... You simply say it ten times in a row... Ten times you whisper... I let go of the fear because I am healthy... Again, you count... You say... I let go of the fear once because I am truly healthy... I let go of the fear twice because I am truly healthy... I let go of the fear three times because I am truly healthy... until you whisper... I let go of the fear ten times because I am truly healthy... and then you feel free from fear and feel that you are healthy...

To wake yourself up again, imagine it starts to hail, and big, cold hailstones hit you... Then you say... Time to go... and then you count energetically to three and open your eyes... It's very easy... So, one more time... To wake yourself up, imagine you're standing in the hail and you say... Time to go – One – Two – Three... and then you're awake and open your eyes... It's very simple, and you can try it out later...

You can do it... You can now use self-hypnosis to let go of fear... You can always let go of the fear of illness on your own and feel healthy... truly healthy... Your deep inner self has learned for you to quickly go into trance with your trigger, and you know how to proceed... Your trigger Iamon brings you into trance, which you deepen with the words I relax and let go... Then follows your suggestion... I let go of the fear because I am truly healthy... and then you imagine cold hailstones and say... Time to go – One – Two – Three...

Hypnosis 10

In our imagination, we sometimes dream ourselves into the most beautiful places we can envision... We simply dive into an inner world of imagination and creativity... a world where we are protected and supported... a world where everything works out and all paths are open to us... And this world truly exists... because imagination and reality are just a blink apart... So today, I invite you to go into this world with yourself... into this land of unlimited possibilities deep within you... the land of dreams... You hear the sound of your breath like the rustling of the wind, which can carry your thoughts away... and with the wind of your breath, you go on a journey into the land of dreams... in this very moment, you arrive there...

The land of dreams lies deep in your imagination, but imagination and reality are just a blink apart... You hear the sound of bubbling water and the music in the background, and with that, you immerse yourself in the idea of being in a completely natural state... The sound of the water and the singing of birds remind you of the sunrise and, with it, the self-evident nature of creation... But in our human existence, not everything is so self-evident, because creation has given us a special gift, free will... Free will is not just the ability to make a decision about what we want, what we will say or do... Free will is also the opportunity open to us to accept our past as it was because we can no longer change it, and even discussing and processing the past cannot influence it anymore... Accepting our own history also means learning from it and then living in our present... with memories that can be painful but can help shape the present... We can choose to let go of wrestling with the past, wishing it had been different... This does not mean, however, that there are no guilty parties or responsibilities or that everything should be forgiven... This message is not known in the land of dreams because the idea of forgiving wrongs suffered would be equivalent to you taking on responsibility or guilt because as humans, we can't help but think in terms of responsibility and accountability... You may forgive, but you don't have to... Forgiveness has nothing to do with your fear of illness, nor with how it can be resolved... The healing path is a different one... You were born a human being, and with that, with the longing to be loved, this is part of being human... But love was not unconditional in your childhood; maybe it never was or never could be... The drama of your life was and is that your feelings were not always allowed to be... What you felt, often no one could or wanted to hear, or only a few... So it happened that to get affection, you often suppressed your feelings as a child... so often and so long until you could no longer really feel them, until there was more and more an unclear feeling inside you that something was wrong... Feelings teach us how we can shape life in the future... Unclear feelings teach us uncertainty and lead to too much building up inside us that we can no longer process properly... because life goes on, flows like the bubbling water you hear in the sounds in the background... But all feelings are still within you, just as they actually were... unaltered and real... They are stored in your body as memories... There are just others on top, those imposed on you or those you chose because you often believed you had to suppress or deny your feelings to protect others... Perhaps you are one of those people who did that even as a child... You are in the land of your dreams and are surrounded by the color gray, which shows you that the confusion and overlap of the many unclear feelings that were not yours have produced your fear of illness... Then you immerse yourself in the color white, which is the counterpart to gray within you and can take on the task of dissolving the gray and providing clarity... In the land of dreams, white is the color of cleansing and clarity and thus the hope for a new inner order of your feelings, which then lets your fear disappear... Then you immerse yourself in the light blue, which for you in the future should be the color of lovingly accepting your history and letting go of the need to change what has happened... What is past, you can and may and should mourn... with all the tears and lamentations that may be necessary, but there can be no reparation for it except for the reparation of your inner emotional order, and for that, there is the land of dreams... Then you are surrounded by the color ochre, which in the land of dreams is the color of recognition, understanding, and learning... and you will recognize, understand, and learn everything that will help you free yourself from fear... Then comes the color silver as the color of truth... It tells you that freedom from fear is possible... and the most precious color is gold, which symbolizes and activates the vitality within you... Gold reminds you that you too are supported by creation and nature... in the land of dreams and in your waking everyday life... Then you immerse yourself in the color red, the color of love and self-love, which allows you to find yourself good and accept yourself, even more so, to love yourself... maybe today or tomorrow or a little bit every day of your life... Self-love helps you the most because it first helps you accept yourself... just as you are... Above all, the red of the dreamland also helps you accept yourself when the fear doesn't fade as quickly as you wish...

You let the colors of the dreamland take effect... Deep within you, they work now and every day and free you from the fear of illness... In the land of dreams, it is enough to be there and do nothing, because the land of dreams takes care of everything necessary for you... But where is the land of dreams?... The land of dreams is the land of your feelings, and therefore it lies deep within you... It has always been there... I'm just telling you about it...

All Titles in the Series

Volume 1: Smoking Cessation
Volume 2: Anxiety and Restlessness
Volume 3: Burnout
Volume 4: Reducing Overweight
Volume 5: Coping with the Past
Volume 6: Suicidal Thoughts and Attempts
Volume 7: Psycho-Oncology
Volume 8: Obsessions and Tics
Volume 9: Self-Confidence and Decision-Making
Volume 10: Grief Work
Volume 11: Psychosomatics
Volume 12: Chronic Pain
Volume 13: Depressive Thoughts
Volume 14: Panic Attacks
Volume 15: Domestic Violence, Victim Support
Volume 16: Post-Traumatic Stress
Volume 17: Exam Anxiety and Stage Fright
Volume 18: Anti-Violence Training, Offender Support
Volume 19: Addiction Tendencies
Volume 20: Social Phobia and Fear of Contact
Volume 21: Nail Biting
Volume 22: Self-Awareness and Self-Love
Volume 23: Teeth Grinding and Night Clenching
Volume 24: Feelings of Guilt
Volume 25: Fear in Crowds
Volume 26: Fear of Flying, Aviophobia
Volume 27: Fear in Enclosed Spaces, Claustrophobia
Volume 28: Tinnitus, Ear Noises
Volume 29: Fear of Heights
Volume 30: Neurodermatitis

Volume 31: Finding Inner Balance
Volume 32: Overcoming Loneliness
Volume 33: Fear of Illness, Hypochondria
Volume 34: Anticipatory Anxiety, Fear of Fear
Volume 35: Jealousy in Relationships
Volume 36: Driving Anxiety
Volume 37: New Start after Separation
Volume 38: Fear of Injections
Volume 39: Heart Anxiety Neurosis
Volume 40: Overcoming Resentment and Anger
Volume 41: Resolving Blockages and Positive Thinking
Volume 42: Stress Reduction, Stress Management
Volume 43: Body Relaxation
Volume 44: Deep Relaxation
Volume 45: Fear of the Dark
Volume 46: Falling Asleep and Staying Asleep
Volume 47: Compulsive Buying
Volume 48: Restless Legs Syndrome
Volume 49: Bulimia
Volume 50: Anorexia
Volume 51: Overcoming Nightmares
Volume 52: Imagined Deformity
Volume 53: Overcoming Distrust, Finding Trust
Volume 54: Processing Failures
Volume 55: Humiliation, Emotional Hurt
Volume 56: Distressing Compassion, Vicarious Suffering
Volume 57: Self-Forgiveness
Volume 58: Self-Awareness, Self-Confidence
Volume 59: Saying No
Volume 60: Assertiveness
Volume 61: Setting Boundaries and Self-Assertion
Volume 62: Decision-Making Ability

Volume 63: Success Orientation
Volume 64: Ruminating, Circular Thinking
Volume 65: Accepting Pregnancy
Volume 66: Birth Preparation
Volume 67: Spiritual Opening
Volume 68: Joy of Life and Inner Lightness
Volume 69: Patience and Inner Peace
Volume 70: Fibromyalgia and Rheumatism
Volume 71: Irritable Bowel Syndrome, Crohn's Disease
Volume 72: Fear of Nausea, Emetophobia
Volume 73: Stuttering and Cluttering, Speech Flow Disorders
Volume 74: Concentration and Knowledge Anchoring
Volume 75: Vitality and Spontaneity
Volume 76: Searching for Meaning and Finding Goals
Volume 77: Life Crises, Life Events
Volume 78: Workaholism, Goal Obsession
Volume 79: Helper Syndrome, Helpless Helpers
Volume 80: Medication Abuse
Volume 81: Gambling Addiction
Volume 82: Internet Addiction, Smartphone Addiction
Volume 83: Hoarding Disorder, Compulsive Collecting
Volume 84: Conspiracy Thoughts, Overvalued Ideas
Volume 85: Fear of Operations and Treatments
Volume 86: Fear of Aging
Volume 87: Travel Anxiety
Volume 88: Anxiety When Urinating, Paruresis
Volume 89: Fear of Intimacy and Togetherness
Volume 90: Fear of Blushing
Volume 91: Coming Out in Homosexuality
Volume 92: Charisma Training
Volume 93: Migraines and Chronic Headaches
Volume 94: Overcoming Allergies, Bronchial Asthma

Volume 95: Normalizing Blood Pressure
Volume 96: Compulsive Perfectionism
Volume 97: Sports Hypnosis, Motivation
Volume 98: Sports Hypnosis, Performance Enhancement
Volume 99: Determination and Focus
Volume 100: Encountering the Inner Child
Volume 101: Cravings, Binge Eating
Volume 102: Stimulating Metabolism
Volume 103: Bipolar Mood Swings
Volume 104: Borderline, Identity Crises
Volume 105: Hypomania, Euphoria, Mania
Volume 106: Restlessness, Agitation
Volume 107: Nervous Breakdown
Volume 108: Adjustment Disorders
Volume 109: Self-Alienation, Depersonalization
Volume 110: Ending Self-Pity
Volume 111: Primary Gain of Illness
Volume 112: Secondary Gain of Illness
Volume 113: Bullying, Victim Support
Volume 114: Letting Go of Envy and Jealousy
Volume 115: Fear of Spiders, Arachnophobia
Volume 116: Fear of Dogs or Cats
Volume 117: Fear of Strangers, Xenophobia
Volume 118: Excessive Worries, Generalized Anxiety
Volume 119: Strengthening Sense of Responsibility
Volume 120: Unrequited Love, Heartache
Volume 121: Work-Life Balance
Volume 122: Letting Go of Unattainable Goals
Volume 123: Allowing and Accepting Help
Volume 124: Letting Go of Adult Children
Volume 125: Tourette Syndrome
Volume 126: Life Changes and New Starts

Volume 127: Accepting Life in a Wheelchair
Volume 128: Understanding and Overcoming Homesickness
Volume 129: Understanding and Overcoming Wanderlust
Volume 130: Dizziness, Meniere's Disease
Volume 131: Overcoming Aggression
Volume 132: Cutting and Self-Harm
Volume 133: Hair Pulling, Trichotillomania
Volume 134: Postpartum Depression
Volume 135: For Relatives of Dementia Patients
Volume 136: Self-Harm, Artificial Disorders
Volume 137: Activating Self-Healing Powers
Volume 138: Preventing Depression Relapse
Volume 139: Reactive Psychoses, Follow-Up
Volume 140: Obsessive Thoughts and Impulses
Volume 141: Compulsive Checking
Volume 142: Compulsive Counting, Symmetry Obsession
Volume 143: Compulsive Washing, Cleanliness Obsession
Volume 144: Compulsive Questioning
Volume 145: Dissociative Paralysis
Volume 146: Phantom Pain
Volume 147: Overcoming Complaining
Volume 148: Hay Fever, Pollen Allergy
Volume 149: Sexual Abuse, Victim Support
Volume 150: Standing Strong Against Sexism, #metoo
Volume 151: Binge Eating
Volume 152: Overcoming Thoughts of Revenge
Volume 153: Detachment from the Aggressor, Stockholm Syndrome
Volume 154: Courage to Separate
Volume 155: Chronic Fatigue, Exhaustion
Volume 156: Fear of the Future, Existential Anxiety
Volume 157: Excessive Worry About Children
Volume 158: Fear of Failure

Volume 159: Ending Distrust and Control
Volume 160: Dejection, Dysphoria
Volume 161: Boreout, Chronic Boredom
Volume 162: Bipolar Disorders, Relapse Prevention
Volume 163: Mania, Relapse Prevention
Volume 164: Nihilism, Feelings of Worthlessness
Volume 165: Thumb Sucking
Volume 166: Being Brave
Volume 167: Being Proud
Volume 168: Overcoming Shyness
Volume 169: Being Able to Delegate Responsibility
Volume 170: Being Able to Show Emotions
Volume 171: Letting Go of Guilt, Victim Support
Volume 172: Processing Guilt, Offender Support
Volume 173: Mood Swings, Cyclothymia
Volume 174: Lack of Drive, Vital Sadness
Volume 175: Hearing Voices with Reality Reference
Volume 176: Confident Communication
Volume 177: Standing Up for Oneself
Volume 178: Taking New Paths
Volume 179: Confident Job Application
Volume 180: No Longer Being Taken Advantage Of
Volume 181: End of Submissiveness
Volume 182: Depressive Numbness
Volume 183: Mood Drops, Affective Incontinence
Volume 184: Mood Instability
Volume 185: Somatoform Disorders
Volume 186: Stomach Ulcer, Psychosomatic
Volume 187: Accepting Amputation
Volume 188: Overcoming and Letting Go of Hatred
Volume 189: Ending Accusations
Volume 190: Allowing Tears, Being Able to Cry

Volume 191: Finding and Sorting Repressed Feelings
Volume 192: Somatoform Pain
Volume 193: Living Autonomously
Volume 194: Anhedonia, Joylessness
Volume 195: Persistent Sadness
Volume 196: Obesity, Food Addiction
Volume 197: Parents of Abused Children
Volume 198: Letting Go and Letting Be
Volume 199: Childhood Sexual Abuse
Volume 200: Fear of Loss

www.ingramcontent.com/pod-product-compliance
Lightning Source LLC
Chambersburg PA
CBHW030504220526
45464CB00006B/2655